THE HEALTHY GUT DIET BOOK

Delicious And Nutrient-Rich Breakfast Recipes For Enhancing Gut Health, Boosting Energy Levels, And Detoxifying Your Body For Chronic Disease Prevention And Weight Loss.

Charlotte Harry

Table of Contents

CHAPTER ONE

UNDERSTANDING THE GUT

The gut, often referred to as the digestive system, plays a crucial role in our overall health. While its primary function is to break down the food we eat, absorb nutrients, and expel waste, the gut's responsibilities extend far beyond digestion. Emerging research highlights the gut's integral role in maintaining a healthy immune system, influencing mental health, and regulating mood. This intricate network of functions is why the gut is often called the "second brain."

Digestion and Nutrient Absorption

The gut is central to the digestive process, breaking down food into smaller molecules that the body can absorb and utilize. The stomach and intestines work together to extract essential nutrients like vitamins, minerals, and amino acids, which are then absorbed into the bloodstream. These nutrients are vital for various bodily functions, including energy production, cell repair, and growth. Any disruption in this process, such as imbalances in gut flora or inflammation, can lead to nutrient deficiencies and associated health problems.

Immune Function

A significant portion of the body's immune system is housed in the gut, particularly within the gut-associated lymphoid tissue (GALT). This tissue contains immune cells that help identify and fight off pathogens that enter the body through food and drink. A healthy gut maintains a balanced environment where beneficial bacteria outnumber harmful ones, thereby supporting immune function. Dysbiosis, an imbalance in gut bacteria, can compromise the immune system, making the body more susceptible to infections and autoimmune diseases.

Mental Health and Mood Regulation

The gut-brain axis is a complex communication network linking the gut and the brain, involving neural, hormonal, and immunological signaling pathways. The gut produces several neurotransmitters, including serotonin, often referred to as the "feel-good" hormone, which plays a critical role in regulating mood and anxiety. In fact, approximately 90% of the body's serotonin is produced in the gut. The vagus nerve, the primary conduit of the gut-brain axis, allows for direct communication between the gut and the brain. This connection explains why gut health can significantly impact mental well-being. Studies have shown that imbalances in gut bacteria can contribute to mental health conditions such as depression and anxiety.

Health Implications of an Unhealthy Gut

An unhealthy gut can manifest in various ways, affecting different aspects of health. Common symptoms of gut imbalance include bloating, gas, diarrhea, and constipation. More severe consequences include chronic conditions like irritable bowel syndrome (IBS) and inflammatory bowel disease (IBD). Additionally, there is growing evidence linking poor gut health to allergies, asthma, and even metabolic disorders like obesity and diabetes. The interplay between gut health and the immune system means that an unhealthy gut can lead to increased inflammation and a weakened immune response.

Anatomy And Functions Of The Gut

The gut is an intricate and essential system that extends from the mouth to the anus, comprising several key components, each with distinct functions crucial to the digestive process and overall health. This system includes the mouth, esophagus, stomach, small intestine, large intestine (colon), and rectum, each playing a vital role in the digestion and absorption of nutrients, as well as the elimination of waste.

The journey of digestion begins in the mouth, where the process of breaking down food starts. Chewing mechanically disintegrates food into smaller pieces, increasing the surface area for enzymes to act upon. Saliva, produced by salivary glands, contains enzymes like amylase that initiate the chemical breakdown of carbohydrates. This mixture of food and saliva, now called a bolus, is swallowed and moves into the esophagus.

The esophagus is a muscular tube that connects the mouth to the stomach. Its primary function is to transport the bolus through peristaltic movements, which are wave-like contractions of the muscles lining the esophagus. This ensures that the food reaches the stomach, regardless of the body's position.

In the stomach, the food undergoes further breakdown. The stomach's muscular walls churn the food, mixing it with gastric juices that contain hydrochloric acid and digestive enzymes, such as pepsin. These substances help to break down proteins into smaller peptides and kill potential pathogens ingested with food. The resulting semi-liquid mixture, called chyme, gradually passes into the small intestine.

The small intestine is the site where most nutrient absorption occurs. It is divided into three sections: the duodenum, jejunum, and ileum. The walls of the small intestine are lined with villi and microvilli, tiny hair-like structures that significantly increase the surface area for absorption. Here, enzymes from the pancreas and bile from the liver further aid in digesting fats, proteins, and carbohydrates. Nutrients and minerals are absorbed through the intestinal walls into the bloodstream, where they are transported to various parts of the body.

Following the small intestine, the large intestine, or colon, plays a crucial role in absorbing water and electrolytes from the remaining indigestible food matter. This process helps to form solid stool. The colon also houses a rich microbiota, which is essential for fermenting undigested carbohydrates, producing certain vitamins, and protecting against harmful bacteria.

Finally, the rectum serves as a temporary storage site for feces before they are expelled from the body through the anus. The process of defecation involves complex coordination of the rectal and anal muscles, controlled by both voluntary and involuntary nervous system mechanisms.

In addition to these mechanical and chemical functions, the gut is intricately connected to the nervous system. Millions of nerve cells, collectively known as the enteric nervous system, are embedded in the gut lining. This "second brain" regulates digestive processes and communicates with the central nervous system, influencing not only digestion but also mood and overall well-being.

Gut Microbiome: An Introduction

The gut microbiome is a vast and complex community of trillions of microorganisms that reside in the digestive tract. This community includes bacteria, viruses, fungi, and other microbes, all of which play a crucial role in various bodily functions. The importance of the gut microbiome extends far beyond digestion, influencing immune function, metabolism, and even mental health.

The diversity and balance of these microorganisms are essential for maintaining health. Beneficial bacteria in the gut aid in the digestion of food, breaking down complex carbohydrates and fibers that the body cannot digest on its own. These bacteria also produce essential vitamins, such as B vitamins and vitamin K, which are vital for energy production and blood clotting, respectively. Additionally, beneficial microbes help protect against harmful bacteria by competing for resources and space, thus preventing infections and maintaining a healthy gut environment.

Several factors can influence the composition and health of the gut microbiome. Diet is a primary factor; a diet rich in fiber, fruits, vegetables, and fermented foods can promote the growth of beneficial bacteria. In contrast, a diet high in processed foods, sugar, and unhealthy fats can lead to a decrease in beneficial bacteria and an increase in harmful bacteria. Antibiotics, while necessary for treating bacterial infections, can also disrupt the balance of the gut microbiome by killing both harmful and beneficial bacteria. This disruption can lead to a state known as dysbiosis, where the imbalance of gut microbes can cause health problems.

Lifestyle factors, such as stress, sleep, and exercise, also play a significant role in shaping the gut microbiome. Chronic stress and lack of sleep can negatively affect the gut microbiome, while regular physical activity has been shown to promote a healthy balance of gut bacteria.

A healthy gut microbiome is linked to numerous health benefits. It enhances digestion, allowing for the efficient absorption of nutrients and the smooth functioning of the digestive system. A balanced microbiome also strengthens the immune system by training it to distinguish between harmful and harmless substances, thus preventing autoimmune reactions and infections. Furthermore, emerging research suggests a strong connection between gut health and mental well-being. The gut-brain axis, a bidirectional communication system between the gut and the brain, indicates that a healthy gut microbiome can positively influence mood, anxiety, and overall mental health.

Conversely, an imbalanced gut microbiome is associated with various health issues. Dysbiosis can contribute to digestive disorders such as irritable bowel syndrome (IBS) and inflammatory bowel disease (IBD). It has also been linked to obesity, metabolic syndrome, and type 2 diabetes due to its role in regulating metabolism and inflammation. Moreover, an unhealthy gut microbiome may influence mental health conditions, including depression and anxiety, through the gut-brain axis.

How The Gut Affects The Immune System

The gut is a major player in the body's immune system, with about 70% of the immune system located within the gut, specifically in the gut-associated lymphoid tissue (GALT). This tissue is a critical component of the immune system, containing a variety of immune cells, such as T cells, B cells, and macrophages, which work together to protect the body from pathogens. The GALT is strategically positioned to monitor and respond to the vast array of antigens and microorganisms that enter the gut through food and other ingested substances.

The gut microbiome, which consists of trillions of microorganisms, including bacteria, viruses, fungi, and protozoa, plays a crucial role in the immune system's functioning. These microorganisms interact closely with the immune cells in the GALT, helping to train the immune system to distinguish between harmful and harmless substances. This interaction is vital for the development of immune tolerance, where the immune system learns to ignore non-threatening substances, such as food proteins and commensal bacteria, while remaining vigilant against pathogens.

A healthy gut microbiome is essential for maintaining the balance of the immune system. The beneficial bacteria in the gut produce various metabolites, such as short-chain fatty acids (SCFAs), which have anti-inflammatory properties and help regulate the activity of immune cells. These metabolites also support the integrity of the gut barrier, preventing harmful substances from crossing into the bloodstream and triggering an immune response.

Disruptions in the gut microbiome, often referred to as dysbiosis, can lead to immune system dysfunction. Dysbiosis can result from factors such as poor diet, stress, antibiotic use, and infections. When the balance of the gut microbiome is disturbed, it can lead to an overactive immune response, contributing to the development of allergies and autoimmune diseases, where the immune system mistakenly attacks the body's own tissues. For example, conditions such as inflammatory bowel disease (IBD), celiac disease, and type 1 diabetes have been linked to dysbiosis and abnormal immune responses in the gut.

Furthermore, dysbiosis can increase susceptibility to infections by weakening the gut barrier and impairing the immune system's ability to respond to pathogens effectively. A compromised gut barrier allows harmful bacteria and toxins to enter the bloodstream, triggering systemic inflammation and potentially leading to infections and other health issues.

Common Gut Disorders And Symptoms

Gut health is a critical aspect of overall well-being, and several common gut disorders can significantly affect quality of life. These disorders include Irritable Bowel Syndrome (IBS), Inflammatory Bowel Disease (IBD), Gastroesophageal

Reflux Disease (GERD), Celiac Disease, and Small Intestinal Bacterial Overgrowth (SIBO). Each condition has unique characteristics and symptoms, but they often share common manifestations such as abdominal pain, bloating, and changes in bowel habits.

Irritable Bowel Syndrome (IBS) is a prevalent functional gastrointestinal disorder. It is primarily characterized by a combination of symptoms, including abdominal pain, bloating, and alterations in bowel habits, such as diarrhea, constipation, or a mixture of both. The exact cause of IBS is unknown, but it is believed to result from a combination of factors, including gut-brain interactions, gastrointestinal motility issues, and heightened sensitivity of the gut. Managing

IBS typically involves dietary modifications, stress management, and sometimes medication.

Inflammatory Bowel Disease (IBD) is an umbrella term for chronic inflammatory conditions of the gastrointestinal tract, including Crohn's disease and ulcerative colitis. Crohn's disease can affect any part of the GI tract from the mouth to the anus, whereas ulcerative colitis is limited to the colon and rectum. Both conditions cause persistent inflammation, leading to symptoms like severe abdominal pain, diarrhea, weight loss, and fatigue. The exact cause of IBD remains unclear, but it is believed to involve an abnormal immune response to gut microbes. Treatment usually includes medication to control inflammation, lifestyle changes, and sometimes surgery.

Gastroesophageal Reflux Disease (GERD) occurs when stomach acid frequently flows back into the esophagus, irritating its lining. This reflux causes symptoms such as heartburn, chest pain, and regurgitation of food or sour liquid. Over time, GERD can lead to more serious health issues, including esophageal inflammation, strictures, and Barrett's esophagus, a condition that can increase the risk of esophageal cancer. Lifestyle modifications, such as avoiding certain foods, eating smaller meals, and not lying down after eating, along with medications, can help manage GERD symptoms.

Celiac Disease is an autoimmune disorder triggered by the ingestion of gluten, a protein found in wheat, barley, and rye. In people with celiac disease, gluten intake leads to damage in the small intestine, specifically the villi, which are essential for nutrient absorption. Symptoms can include diarrhea, weight loss, fatigue, and anemia. The only effective treatment for celiac disease is a strict gluten-free diet, which helps to heal intestinal damage and prevent further complications.

Small Intestinal Bacterial Overgrowth (SIBO) involves an abnormal increase in the number of bacteria in the small intestine. This overgrowth can interfere with nutrient absorption and lead to symptoms like bloating, diarrhea, and malabsorption. SIBO can result from various underlying conditions, such as motility disorders, anatomical abnormalities, or immune deficiencies. Treatment often involves antibiotics to reduce bacterial overgrowth, dietary changes, and addressing any underlying conditions.

Symptoms of these gut disorders can vary widely but commonly include abdominal pain, bloating, gas, diarrhea, constipation, and changes in appetite. Proper diagnosis and management of gut disorders are essential for maintaining overall health and well-being, as these conditions can significantly impact daily life and long-term health outcomes. Identifying the specific disorder and implementing appropriate treatments can help alleviate symptoms and improve quality of life.

CHAPTER TWO

THE GUT-BRAIN CONNECTION

The Science Behind The Gut-Brain Axis

The gut-brain axis represents a sophisticated communication network linking the gastrointestinal (GI) system with the brain. This connection is bidirectional, allowing for a dynamic exchange of information whereby the brain can influence gut function and the gut can affect brain activity. Central to this network is the enteric nervous system (ENS), often called the "second brain," which boasts around 100 million neurons. These neurons interact with the central nervous system (CNS) via various channels, including the vagus nerve, hormones, and immune system signals.

One of the most significant elements of the gut-brain axis is the gut microbiota. This diverse community of microorganisms resides in the intestines and plays an essential role in human health. The microbiota produces a variety of neurotransmitters, such as serotonin and dopamine, which are vital for mood regulation, cognitive functions, and digestive processes. For instance, approximately 90% of the body's serotonin is produced in the gut, highlighting the significant role the gut plays in regulating mood and mental well-being.

The vagus nerve acts as a primary conduit for the gut-brain communication. This long nerve runs from the brainstem to the abdomen, transmitting signals between the gut and the brain. Through this pathway, the gut can send information about the state of the digestive system to the brain, influencing stress responses, mood, and overall mental health. Conversely, the brain can send signals that impact gut motility, enzyme secretion, and the permeability of the gut lining.

Disruptions in the gut microbiota, often termed dysbiosis, can have far-reaching consequences. Dysbiosis can result from factors such as poor diet, chronic stress, infections, or antibiotic use. When the balance of gut bacteria is disturbed, it can lead to increased inflammation and alterations in neurotransmitter production. These changes are associated with various mental health conditions, including anxiety and depression. For example, individuals with irritable bowel syndrome (IBS) often experience comorbid psychological symptoms, underscoring the tight link between gut health and mental state.

Additionally, the gut-brain axis influences cognitive functions and brain development. Emerging research suggests that gut bacteria can impact the development of the blood-brain barrier, neurogenesis, and myelination of neurons. These processes are crucial for maintaining brain health and function throughout life.

How Emotions Affect Gut Health

Emotions significantly influence gut health, a connection rooted in the intricate communication between the brain and the gastrointestinal system, often referred to as the gut-brain axis. This bidirectional relationship means that when you experience strong emotions such as anxiety, fear, or excitement, your brain sends signals to your gut, impacting its functionality. This phenomenon explains why you might feel butterflies in your stomach before a significant event or suffer from digestive issues during periods of heightened stress.

Negative emotions, especially chronic stress, can severely affect gut health, leading to a condition commonly known as "leaky gut." The gut lining is designed to be selectively permeable, allowing essential nutrients to pass into the bloodstream while keeping harmful substances out. However, under chronic stress, the gut lining can become excessively permeable. This increased permeability means that undigested food particles, toxins, and microbes can pass through the gut wall into the bloodstream, triggering inflammation and contributing to various health issues. Conditions such as irritable bowel syndrome (IBS), food intolerances, and autoimmune diseases are often linked to leaky gut syndrome, illustrating the profound impact of emotional well-being on gut health.

Moreover, stress and negative emotions can disrupt the delicate balance of the gut microbiota, the diverse community of bacteria residing in the intestines. The gut microbiota plays a crucial role in digestion, immune function, and overall health. Chronic stress has been shown to reduce the diversity of gut bacteria, leading to an imbalance known as dysbiosis. Dysbiosis is associated with several health problems, including obesity, autoimmune diseases, and mental health disorders such as anxiety and depression. The reduced diversity and imbalance of gut bacteria can impair the gut's ability to function correctly, further exacerbating health issues.

Research has demonstrated that the gut microbiota can influence the central nervous system, impacting mood and behavior. This means that not only can emotions affect gut health, but gut health can also influence emotions, creating a feedback loop. For instance, certain gut bacteria produce neurotransmitters like serotonin and dopamine, which play a critical role in regulating mood. An imbalance in these bacteria can lead to mood disorders, highlighting the importance of maintaining a healthy gut for emotional well-being.

The Impact Of Stress On The Gut

Stress significantly impacts the gut, influencing both its functionality and overall health. When a person experiences stress, the body activates the "fight or flight" response, releasing stress hormones such as cortisol and adrenaline. These hormones prepare the body to respond to perceived threats, but they also affect gut motility. Depending on the individual, this can result in either a slowing down or speeding up of the digestive process, leading to symptoms such as diarrhea, constipation, and abdominal pain.

The gut-brain axis, a bidirectional communication system between the central nervous system and the gastrointestinal tract, plays a crucial role in this process. Stress can disrupt this axis, leading to a variety of gastrointestinal symptoms. For instance, stress-induced changes in gut motility and secretion can alter the balance of gut microbiota, further contributing to digestive issues.

People with pre-existing gut conditions, like irritable bowel syndrome (IBS), often find that their symptoms worsen during periods of stress. IBS is a chronic condition characterized by abdominal pain, bloating, and altered bowel habits. Stress can increase the sensitivity of the gut, making it more responsive to pain and discomfort. This heightened sensitivity is due to the interaction between stress hormones and the enteric nervous system, which controls gastrointestinal function. The result is an exacerbation of IBS symptoms, creating a vicious cycle where stress and gut issues feed into each other.

Moreover, stress impacts the gut's immune function. The gut is home to a significant portion of the body's immune cells, and a well-functioning immune system is vital for maintaining gut health. Chronic stress can weaken the immune system, making it less effective at defending against pathogens. This increased susceptibility can lead to infections and inflammation within the gut. Inflammation, in turn, can damage the gut lining, leading to conditions like leaky gut syndrome, where the intestinal barrier becomes permeable and allows harmful substances to enter the bloodstream.

Furthermore, stress can alter the gut microbiome, the community of microorganisms living in the intestines. A healthy microbiome is essential for digestion, nutrient absorption, and immune function. Stress can disrupt this delicate balance, reducing the diversity of gut bacteria and allowing harmful bacteria to proliferate. This imbalance, known as dysbiosis, can contribute to various health problems, including digestive disorders, obesity, and mental health issues.

Strategies For Managing Stress And Anxiety

Managing stress and anxiety is crucial for maintaining gut health, as the two are closely linked through the gut-brain axis. Implementing effective strategies to manage these issues can lead to significant improvements in overall well-being and gut function.

Mindfulness and Meditation

Mindfulness and meditation practices are powerful tools for stress reduction. By focusing on the present moment and cultivating a state of non-judgmental awareness, mindfulness can significantly lower stress levels. Meditation techniques, such as deep breathing, progressive muscle relaxation, and guided imagery, promote relaxation and help manage negative emotions. These practices encourage a calmer mind, which positively impacts gut health by reducing the production of stress hormones that can disrupt digestive function.

Exercise

Regular physical activity is another effective way to manage stress and anxiety.

Exercise releases endorphins, which are natural mood elevators and stress relievers. Activities like walking, running, yoga, or even dancing can significantly reduce stress levels. Moreover, exercise promotes healthy gut motility, which is essential for preventing issues like constipation. It also supports a balanced gut microbiota, which is crucial for overall digestive health. Engaging in physical activity regularly can help maintain a healthy gut environment, thereby improving both mental and physical health.

Healthy Diet

A balanced diet plays a pivotal role in managing stress and supporting gut health. Consuming foods rich in fiber, probiotics, and prebiotics can enhance gut health and mitigate the adverse effects of stress.

Probiotic foods like yogurt, kefir, and sauerkraut introduce beneficial bacteria to the gut, promoting a healthy microbiome. Prebiotics, found in foods like whole grains, bananas, and asparagus, feed these beneficial bacteria, helping them thrive. Fiber-rich foods aid in digestion and prevent gastrointestinal problems that can be exacerbated by stress. Thus, a diet rich in these nutrients can help manage stress and maintain a healthy gut.

Adequate Sleep

Ensuring adequate sleep is essential for both stress management and gut health. Lack of sleep can increase stress levels and negatively impact the gut microbiota. Poor sleep patterns are associated with increased inflammation and dysbiosis, which is an imbalance in the gut bacteria.

Establishing a regular sleep routine and creating a conducive sleep environment can help improve sleep quality. Techniques like limiting screen time before bed, maintaining a cool and dark bedroom, and practicing relaxation exercises can promote better sleep. Improved sleep helps reduce stress and supports a healthy gut microbiome.

Therapy and Support

Seeking therapy and support is another effective strategy for managing stress and anxiety. Speaking with a therapist can provide valuable insights and coping strategies. Cognitive-behavioral therapy (CBT) is particularly effective in helping individuals identify and change negative thought patterns and behaviors. Joining support groups can also offer emotional support and practical advice from others experiencing similar issues. Engaging in therapy and support networks can significantly improve stress management, which in turn, positively impacts gut health.

The Role Of Sleep In Gut Health

Sleep plays a crucial role in maintaining overall health, including the well-being of the gut. During sleep, the body undergoes various repair and maintenance processes essential for optimal functioning, with the gut being a significant area of focus. Ensuring adequate sleep helps regulate the production of stress hormones, which can protect the gut from the harmful effects of chronic stress.

The relationship between sleep and gut health is profound and complex. The gut is home to a diverse community of bacteria known as the gut microbiota, which plays a vital role in digestion, immune function, and mental health. Studies have shown that poor sleep quality or insufficient sleep can lead to alterations in the composition of these gut bacteria, a condition known as dysbiosis. Dysbiosis can disrupt digestion, weaken the immune system, and negatively impact mental health, leading to issues such as anxiety and depression.

One of the primary ways sleep affects the gut is through the regulation of the circadian rhythm, the body's internal clock that controls the sleep-wake cycle. The gut microbiota also follows a circadian rhythm, and disruptions in sleep can misalign this natural cycle, causing imbalances in gut bacteria. These imbalances can impair the gut's ability to function correctly, leading to symptoms such as bloating, constipation, and diarrhea. Additionally, the gut-brain axis, a bidirectional communication system between the gut and the brain, is heavily influenced by sleep. Poor sleep can impair this communication, leading to increased inflammation and a heightened stress response, both of which can negatively affect gut health.

To promote better sleep and, consequently, better gut health, it is essential to establish a regular sleep schedule. Going to bed and waking up at the same time every day helps regulate the body's internal clock and enhances sleep quality. Creating a relaxing bedtime routine can also prepare the body for sleep. Activities such as reading, taking a warm bath, or practicing meditation can signal the body that it is time to wind down.

Avoiding stimulants like caffeine and electronic devices before bed is also crucial. Caffeine can interfere with the ability to fall asleep, while the blue light emitted by electronic devices can suppress the production of melatonin, the hormone responsible for regulating sleep. Additionally, ensuring a comfortable sleep environment can significantly improve sleep quality. A dark, quiet, and cool room can create an ideal setting for restful sleep. Investing in a comfortable mattress and pillows, as well as using blackout curtains and white noise machines, can further enhance the sleep environment.

CHAPTER THREE

GUT-FRIENDLY FOODS

The Importance Of Fiber

Fiber is a crucial component of a healthy diet, playing a vital role in maintaining gut health and overall well-being. There are two primary types of dietary fiber: soluble and insoluble. Understanding the differences between these two types and their respective benefits can help in making informed dietary choices.

Soluble Fiber:

Soluble fiber dissolves in water to form a gel-like substance that can slow down digestion. This type of fiber is instrumental in regulating blood sugar levels and improving the absorption of essential nutrients. By delaying the digestion and absorption of carbohydrates, soluble fiber helps to prevent spikes in blood sugar, which is particularly beneficial for individuals with diabetes or those managing their weight. Additionally, soluble fiber can help lower cholesterol levels by binding to cholesterol particles in the digestive system and removing them from the body before they are absorbed into the bloodstream.

Common sources of soluble fiber include oats, beans, lentils, apples, and citrus fruits. Incorporating these foods into your diet can help you achieve the recommended daily intake of fiber, which varies based on age and sex but generally ranges from 25 to 38 grams per day. For example, starting your day with a bowl of oatmeal topped with sliced apples or incorporating beans into your salads and soups are simple ways to boost your soluble fiber intake.

Insoluble Fiber:

In contrast, insoluble fiber does not dissolve in water and adds bulk to the stool, which helps food pass more quickly through the digestive tract. This type of fiber is essential for preventing constipation and promoting regular bowel movements. By increasing the bulk and softness of the stool, insoluble fiber makes it easier for waste to move through the intestines and be expelled from the body. This process helps to maintain bowel health and prevent digestive disorders such as diverticulitis and hemorrhoids.

Whole grains, nuts, seeds, and vegetables like broccoli, carrots, and cauliflower are excellent sources of insoluble fiber. Integrating these foods into your daily meals can significantly enhance your digestive health. For instance, choosing whole grain bread over refined bread or snacking on a handful of nuts instead of processed snacks are effective strategies to increase your insoluble fiber consumption.

Gut Microbiome and Overall Health:

Including a variety of fiber-rich foods in your diet supports a diverse and healthy gut microbiome, which is essential for optimal digestive health. The gut microbiome consists of trillions of bacteria and other microorganisms that reside in the digestive tract. These microorganisms play a crucial role in digestion, immune function, and even mental health. A diet rich in both soluble and insoluble fiber provides the necessary nutrients for these beneficial bacteria to thrive, promoting a balanced and healthy gut environment.

Probiotics And Prebiotics

Probiotics and prebiotics play crucial roles in maintaining a balanced gut microbiome, fostering a symbiotic relationship that is essential for overall health. Probiotics are live beneficial bacteria that reside in the digestive system, helping to keep harmful bacteria in check and supporting various bodily functions. On the other hand, prebiotics are non-digestible fibers that serve as food for these beneficial bacteria, promoting their growth and activity.

Probiotic-rich foods are an excellent way to introduce beneficial bacteria into the gut. Common sources include yogurt, kefir, sauerkraut, kimchi, miso, and tempeh.

These foods undergo a fermentation process that encourages the growth of probiotics. Regular consumption of these foods can improve digestion by enhancing the breakdown of food and absorption of nutrients. Moreover, probiotics boost the immune system by reinforcing the gut barrier against pathogens and stimulating the production of antibodies. Emerging research also suggests a link between probiotics and mental health, as the gut microbiome communicates with the brain through the gut-brain axis, potentially influencing mood and cognitive function.

Prebiotics, found in foods such as garlic, onions, leeks, asparagus, bananas, and whole grains, play an equally important role. These fibers pass through the digestive system undigested until they reach the colon, where they are fermented by the gut bacteria. This fermentation process produces short-chain fatty acids, which serve as an energy source for the colon cells and help maintain the integrity of the gut lining. By nourishing the probiotics, prebiotics ensure these beneficial bacteria thrive, promoting a balanced and healthy gut environment.

The interplay between probiotics and prebiotics is essential for optimal gut health. When both are consumed regularly, they create a synergistic effect that enhances the growth and activity of beneficial bacteria, leading to a healthier and more resilient gut microbiome. This balance can help prevent digestive disorders such as irritable bowel syndrome (IBS) and inflammatory bowel disease

(IBD), reduce the risk of infections, and improve overall health.

Incorporating a variety of probiotic and prebiotic foods into your diet is a practical and effective way to support gut health. For example, starting the day with a breakfast that includes yogurt topped with bananas and whole grains, or incorporating garlic and onions into savory dishes, can provide a balanced intake of both probiotics and prebiotics.

Fermented Foods And Their Benefits

Fermented foods have been celebrated for their health benefits and enjoyed across different cultures for centuries. The fermentation process involves the transformation of sugars in food by bacteria and yeast, which not only helps preserve the food but also significantly enhances its nutritional value.

One of the key benefits of fermented foods is their high probiotic content. Probiotics are live microorganisms that, when consumed in adequate amounts, confer health benefits to the host, primarily by improving gut health. Fermented foods such as yogurt, kefir, sauerkraut, kimchi, miso, and kombucha are rich in these beneficial bacteria.

Yogurt and kefir, for example, are dairy products that have undergone fermentation with specific bacterial cultures. These products are well-known for their probiotic properties, which help maintain a healthy balance of gut bacteria. This balance is crucial for efficient digestion and absorption of nutrients, and it also plays a role in bolstering the immune system. Regular consumption of yogurt and kefir can help alleviate symptoms of lactose intolerance, as the fermentation process breaks down lactose, making these foods easier to digest.

Sauerkraut and kimchi, both made from fermented cabbage, are also excellent sources of probiotics. Sauerkraut, a staple in German cuisine, and kimchi, a Korean delicacy, offer not only probiotic benefits but also a high content of vitamins C and K, and fiber. These nutrients support overall digestive health and help reduce inflammation, a common underlying factor in many chronic diseases.

Miso, a fermented soybean paste, is a fundamental ingredient in Japanese cuisine. It is rich in essential minerals and provides a good source of various B vitamins, vitamins E, K, and folic acid. The fermentation process in miso production also generates isoflavones and saponins, which are compounds known for their antioxidant and anti-inflammatory properties.

Kombucha, a fermented tea, has gained popularity for its potential health benefits, including improved digestion and increased energy levels. This effervescent drink is made by fermenting sweetened tea with a symbiotic culture of bacteria and yeast (SCOBY). Kombucha contains probiotics, antioxidants, and polyphenols that contribute to overall health.

Incorporating a variety of fermented foods into your diet can profoundly impact your gut microbiome. The gut microbiome is a complex community of microorganisms living in the digestive tract, and its balance is essential for overall health. A healthy gut microbiome can improve digestion, enhance immune function, and reduce the risk of many chronic diseases, including inflammatory bowel disease, obesity, and even certain mental health conditions.

Anti-Inflammatory Foods

Chronic inflammation in the gut is a significant factor contributing to various digestive disorders, including irritable bowel syndrome (IBS), Crohn's disease, and ulcerative colitis. This persistent inflammation can also be linked to broader health issues, such as autoimmune diseases and cardiovascular problems. One effective way to combat this inflammation is through the incorporation of anti-inflammatory foods into your diet.

Among the most potent anti-inflammatory foods are fatty fish, particularly salmon, mackerel, and sardines. These fish are rich in omega-3 fatty acids, which have been extensively studied for their ability to reduce inflammation in the body. Omega-3s play a crucial role in the production of anti-inflammatory compounds, thereby helping to lower inflammatory markers in the bloodstream and support overall gut health.

In addition to fatty fish, a variety of fruits and vegetables can also contribute to reducing inflammation. Berries, such as blueberries, strawberries, and raspberries, are particularly high in antioxidants called flavonoids, which help combat oxidative stress and inflammation. Leafy greens like spinach, kale, and Swiss chard are also excellent choices, as they are rich in vitamins, minerals, and phytonutrients that promote health and healing.

Nuts and seeds, including walnuts, flaxseeds, and chia seeds, are another essential group of anti-inflammatory foods. They provide healthy fats, fiber, and protein, which contribute to satiety and overall health. Olive oil, particularly extra virgin olive oil, is another powerful anti-inflammatory food, thanks to its high content of monounsaturated fats and antioxidants. Regular use of olive oil in cooking and dressings can promote heart health and reduce inflammation.

Turmeric, a spice commonly used in various cuisines, is particularly noteworthy for its active compound, curcumin. Curcumin is renowned for its strong anti-inflammatory properties and has been the subject of many studies highlighting its potential health benefits. Adding turmeric to meals can enhance flavor while providing a natural means of supporting gut health and reducing inflammation.

Foods To Avoid For A Healthy Gut

Maintaining a healthy gut is crucial for overall well-being, and while certain foods can enhance gut health, others can have detrimental effects. It's important to be mindful of what you consume, especially when it comes to your gut microbiome. Here are some foods to limit or avoid for optimal gut health.

1. Highly Processed Foods

Processed foods are often loaded with additives, preservatives, and unhealthy fats. These ingredients can disrupt the balance of gut bacteria, leading to digestive issues and inflammation. Common processed items include packaged snacks, fast food, and ready-to-eat meals. Instead, focus on whole foods like fruits, vegetables, lean proteins, and whole grains to nourish your gut.

2. Refined Sugars

Refined sugars, found in sugary drinks, candies, and baked goods, can promote the growth of harmful bacteria and yeast in the gut. This imbalance can contribute to conditions like leaky gut syndrome, which allows toxins to enter the bloodstream, potentially leading to various health issues. Opt for natural sweeteners like honey or fruit, and be mindful of your sugar intake.

3. Artificial Sweeteners

Although often used as a low-calorie alternative, artificial sweeteners can negatively affect gut health. Research suggests that they may alter gut microbiota composition, leading to increased inflammation and potential metabolic issues. Consider using natural sweeteners or reducing overall sweetness in your diet.

4. Alcohol

Alcohol can irritate the gut lining, impairing the protective barrier and disrupting the microbiome's balance. While moderate consumption may be acceptable for some, excessive drinking can lead to significant gut health problems, including gut permeability and inflammation. Limiting alcohol intake can be beneficial for maintaining gut integrity.

5. Caffeine

Caffeine, found in coffee, tea, and energy drinks, can also irritate the gut lining in some individuals. It may lead to increased acidity and digestive discomfort, especially for those with sensitivities. If you notice adverse effects, consider moderating your caffeine consumption.

6. Common Food Intolerances

Many people experience food intolerances that can negatively impact gut health. Common offenders include gluten, dairy, and certain fermentable carbohydrates (FODMAPs). If you suspect you have an intolerance, it's wise to consult a healthcare professional for testing and dietary guidance.

CHAPTER FOUR
CREATING A GUT-HEALTHY DIET PLAN

Assessing Your Current Diet

Starting a journey toward a gut-healthy diet begins with a thorough assessment of your current eating habits. One effective way to gain insight into your diet is to keep a food diary for a week. This practice involves meticulously recording everything you consume, from meals to snacks, and even beverages. As you document your intake, pay close attention to the types of foods you eat, their portion sizes, and your overall eating patterns.

Start by evaluating the quality of your food choices. Are you incorporating a variety of fruits, vegetables, whole grains, and lean proteins into your meals? These foods are rich in nutrients and fiber, which are vital for maintaining gut health. Fiber, in particular, plays a crucial role in promoting healthy digestion and fostering a balanced gut microbiome. On the other hand, take note of your consumption of processed foods, sugary snacks, and high amounts of dairy. These items can often lead to inflammation and may contribute to digestive issues.

After a week of tracking, it's time to analyze your findings. Identify areas where you can make improvements. For instance, if you notice a lack of fruits and vegetables in your diet, consider integrating more of these into your meals and snacks. A diverse range of produce not only provides essential vitamins and minerals but also supports the growth of beneficial gut bacteria.

It's also essential to reflect on how you feel after eating. Pay attention to any discomfort you experience, such as bloating, gas, or fatigue. These symptoms may signal that certain foods do not agree with your digestive system. Perhaps you find that dairy products cause discomfort, or maybe you feel sluggish after consuming high-sugar snacks. Identifying these patterns can help you tailor your diet to better suit your body's needs.

Building A Balanced Meal Plan

Creating a balanced meal plan is essential for promoting gut health and overall well-being. A well-rounded diet should incorporate a variety of foods that nourish beneficial gut bacteria and support digestion. Key to this approach is including plenty of fiber-rich foods, such as fruits, vegetables, legumes, and whole grains. Fiber serves as a prebiotic, feeding the beneficial bacteria in your gut, which can enhance digestion and improve gut function.

In addition to fiber, it's important to include fermented foods in your diet. These foods, which include yogurt, kefir, sauerkraut, kimchi, and kombucha, are rich in probiotics. Probiotics are live microorganisms that can help balance gut flora, potentially improving immune function and promoting overall health. Incorporating a mix of these fermented foods into your meals can have a positive impact on your gut microbiome.

Healthy fats also play a vital role in a balanced meal plan. They are crucial for the absorption of fat-soluble vitamins and overall health. Good sources of healthy fats include avocados, nuts, seeds, and olive oil. These fats not only contribute to nutrient absorption but also help maintain satiety and support heart health.

To effectively build a balanced meal plan, consider the following framework for daily meals:

Breakfast: Kickstart your day with a fiber-rich meal, such as oatmeal topped with fresh berries and a sprinkle of nuts. This combination provides a hearty dose of fiber, antioxidants, and healthy fats, setting a positive tone for your day.

Lunch: For lunch, opt for a vibrant salad filled with mixed greens and an array of colorful vegetables. Add a lean protein source, like grilled chicken or chickpeas, and dress it with a vinaigrette made from olive oil. This meal is not only nutritious but also satisfying.

Dinner: Aim for a balanced dinner by creating a plate that includes a portion of lean protein, such as fish or tofu, steamed vegetables, and a whole grain like quinoa or brown rice. This combination provides essential nutrients and keeps your gut health in check.

Snacks: Throughout the day, choose healthy snacks to maintain energy levels and support gut health. Fresh fruits, crunchy veggies with hummus, or a small handful of nuts are great options that contribute to your overall fiber intake.

Sample Meal Plans For Different Lifestyles

Individuals have varying lifestyles and dietary needs, which can influence their meal choices. Here are three thoughtfully crafted meal plans designed for busy professionals, those with an active lifestyle, and families seeking nutritious options. Each plan focuses on convenience, health, and taste, ensuring that every meal supports the lifestyle it caters to.

Busy Professional:

For the busy professional juggling work commitments, convenience and nutrition are key. Breakfast might start with Greek yogurt topped with honey and granola, providing a quick source of protein and healthy carbohydrates. For lunch, a whole grain wrap filled with turkey, fresh spinach, and creamy avocado offers a satisfying meal that's easy to prepare and pack. As the day winds down, dinner could feature a flavorful stir-fried tofu dish, bursting with colorful mixed vegetables and served over brown rice, creating a wholesome and filling end to the day. Healthy snacks like almonds and a banana are perfect for keeping energy levels up throughout busy workdays.

Active Lifestyle:

Individuals with an active lifestyle require meals that support their energy needs. A refreshing smoothie made with spinach, banana, protein powder, and almond milk makes for an energizing breakfast, packed with nutrients and easily digestible. Lunch could consist of a vibrant quinoa salad tossed with black beans, sweet corn, and diced bell peppers, offering a blend of protein and fiber. For dinner, grilled salmon paired with roasted sweet potatoes and steamed broccoli provides a rich source of omega-3 fatty acids and complex carbohydrates, essential for recovery after a day filled with activity. On-the-go snacks, like energy bars or trail mix, help sustain energy and keep hunger at bay.

Family-Friendly:

For families, meals need to be both nutritious and appealing to all ages. Breakfast might include whole grain pancakes, served with fresh fruit and a drizzle of maple syrup, turning the first meal of the day into a delightful experience. Lunch can be simple yet tasty, with turkey and cheese sandwiches on whole grain bread accompanied by crunchy carrot sticks. Dinner is often a time for gathering, and baked chicken with a medley of roasted vegetables and a side of brown rice makes for a nutritious and satisfying family meal. Snacks such as yogurt with granola or apple slices paired with peanut butter offer healthy options that are easy to prepare and popular among kids.

Shopping Guide For Gut-Friendly Foods

Shopping for gut-friendly foods can be a rewarding experience, especially when you know which categories to prioritize. A healthy gut is essential for overall well-being, and incorporating a variety of foods can help support gut health. Here's a comprehensive guide to help you navigate your grocery shopping for gut-friendly options.

Fruits and Vegetables

Start by filling your cart with a colorful array of fruits and vegetables. Diverse colors often signify a range of nutrients and antioxidants that are beneficial for gut health. High-fiber options, such as apples, pears, berries, broccoli, and leafy greens, are particularly important as they promote healthy digestion and regularity. Aim for organic produce when possible, as it tends to have fewer pesticides and higher nutrient levels.

Whole Grains

When it comes to grains, opt for whole grains rather than refined options. Whole grains retain their bran, germ, and endosperm, making them richer in fiber and nutrients. Good choices include oats, quinoa, brown rice, and whole grain bread or pasta. These grains not only provide energy but also support the growth of beneficial gut bacteria.

Proteins

Incorporating a variety of protein sources is essential for gut health. Lean meats, fish, and eggs are excellent choices, but don't overlook plant-based options. Legumes such as lentils, chickpeas, and beans are not only high in protein but also rich in fiber. Additionally, plant-based proteins like tofu and tempeh offer gut-friendly benefits while being versatile ingredients for many recipes.

Healthy Fats

Healthy fats play a crucial role in overall health, including gut function. Incorporate sources like avocados, nuts, seeds, and olive oil into your meals. These fats help reduce inflammation and support the absorption of fat-soluble vitamins. They also contribute to a feeling of fullness, which can prevent overeating.

Fermented Foods

Fermented foods are particularly beneficial for gut health due to their probiotic content. Probiotics are live bacteria that can help balance your gut microbiome. Include foods like yogurt, kefir, sauerkraut, kimchi, and kombucha in your diet. These items not only add flavor and variety but also support digestive health.

Meal Prep Tips And Tricks

Meal prepping can be a game changer when it comes to maintaining a gut-healthy diet. By dedicating some time each week to prepare meals in advance, you set yourself up for success, making it easier to stick to your nutrition goals. Here are some effective tips to streamline your meal prep process:

1. Plan Ahead: One of the most important aspects of meal prepping is planning. Choose a day each week to sit down and outline your meals. This could be Sunday or any day that fits your schedule. Write down a detailed grocery list based on your planned meals. This not only saves you time during your shopping trip but also minimizes impulse buys that can derail your healthy eating efforts.

2. Batch Cooking: Batch cooking is an efficient way to prepare large quantities of staple foods that can serve as the foundation for multiple meals. Think grains like quinoa, brown rice, or farro, legumes such as lentils or chickpeas, and hearty soups. Cook these in bulk and portion them out for the week. This not only saves time but also ensures you always have nutritious options ready to go.

3. Use Containers: Investing in good-quality, reusable containers can make a world of difference in your meal prep routine. Look for containers that are microwave-safe, dishwasher-friendly, and designed for portion control. Having a variety of sizes on hand allows you to store meals, snacks, and even pre-chopped

ingredients conveniently, making it easy to grab and go.

4. Prep Snacks: Healthy snacking is crucial for keeping your energy levels stable and avoiding unhealthy choices when hunger strikes. Prepare nutritious snacks in advance, such as cut-up vegetables, hummus, nuts, or yogurt. Store these in grab-and-go containers, so they're easily accessible throughout the week. This proactive approach can help curb cravings and keep your gut happy.

5. Stay Flexible: While planning and prepping are essential, it's equally important to remain flexible. Life can be unpredictable, and sometimes your schedule may change. Allow for adjustments in your meal plan as needed. The goal is to enjoy the process and listen

to your body's needs. If a meal doesn't sound appealing on a particular day, swap it out for something else you have prepared.

CHAPTER FIVE

RECIPES FOR GUT HEALTH

Breakfast Recipes

Overnight Oats with Chia Seeds

Ingredients:

1.   1 cup rolled oats

2.   2 cups almond milk (or any preferred milk)

3.   2 tablespoons chia seeds

4.   1 tablespoon honey or maple syrup

5.   Fresh fruits (e.g., berries, banana) for topping

Instructions:

1.   In a bowl or jar, combine the rolled oats, almond milk, chia seeds, and sweetener.

2.   Stir the mixture well to ensure that the chia seeds are evenly distributed and not clumped together.

3.   Cover the bowl or jar and refrigerate it overnight. This allows the oats and chia seeds to absorb the milk and expand, creating a thick, pudding-like consistency.

4.   In the morning, give the mixture another good stir. The oats and chia seeds should be soft and well-incorporated with the milk.

5.   Top the oats with fresh fruits of your choice. Berries, sliced banana, or even a handful of nuts can add flavor, texture, and nutritional value.

6.   Enjoy your overnight oats as a quick, nutritious breakfast that is ready as soon as you wake up.

Overnight oats are a perfect make-ahead breakfast, saving you time in the morning while still providing a nutritious start to your day. The combination of rolled oats and chia seeds offers a good source of fiber and protein, keeping you full and satisfied. Almond milk keeps it dairy-free, and the addition of honey or maple syrup adds just the right amount of sweetness without being overpowering.

Greek Yogurt Parfait

Ingredients:

1.   1 cup plain Greek yogurt

2.   ½ cup granola (preferably low-sugar)

3.   1 cup mixed berries

4.   1 tablespoon flaxseeds

Instructions:

1.   In a tall glass or a bowl, begin by adding a layer of Greek yogurt. Greek yogurt is rich in protein and probiotics, which are great for your gut health.

2.   Next, add a layer of granola. Opt for low-sugar granola to keep the parfait healthy and nutritious. Granola adds a delightful crunch to the creamy yogurt.

3.   Add a layer of mixed berries. Berries such as strawberries, blueberries, and raspberries are packed with antioxidants, vitamins, and minerals.

4.   Continue layering with another portion of Greek yogurt, followed by more granola and berries if your glass or bowl allows. The idea is to have multiple layers

to enjoy a bit of each ingredient in every bite.

5.   Finally, sprinkle a tablespoon of flaxseeds on top. Flaxseeds are a great source of omega-3 fatty acids and fiber, adding even more nutritional value to your parfait.

6.   Serve immediately and enjoy your Greek Yogurt Parfait.

This Greek Yogurt Parfait is not only quick and easy to assemble but also provides a balanced breakfast that includes protein, healthy fats, fiber, and a variety of essential nutrients. It's perfect for busy mornings or as a refreshing snack any time of the day. The combination of creamy yogurt, crunchy granola, and juicy berries makes each bite a delight.

Quinoa Salad with Fermented Vegetables

Ingredients:

1. 1 cup cooked quinoa

2. 1 cup mixed greens

3. ½ cup fermented vegetables (e.g., sauerkraut, kimchi)

4. ¼ cup diced cucumber

5. ¼ cup cherry tomatoes, halved

6. Olive oil and lemon juice for dressing

Instructions:

Start by cooking the quinoa according to package instructions. Once cooked, let it cool to room temperature. In a large mixing bowl, combine the cooked quinoa with a cup of mixed greens, which can include spinach, arugula, or any other leafy greens you prefer. Next, add half a cup of your favorite fermented vegetables. Sauerkraut and kimchi are excellent choices due to their tangy flavor and probiotic benefits. Then, incorporate a quarter cup of diced cucumber for a refreshing crunch, and a quarter cup of halved cherry tomatoes for a burst of sweetness and color.

For the dressing, drizzle the salad with a generous amount of olive oil and freshly squeezed lemon juice. This simple yet flavorful dressing enhances the natural taste of the ingredients without overpowering them. Toss the salad gently to ensure all components are well mixed and evenly coated with the dressing. Serve immediately for a nutritious, gut-friendly lunch that's rich in fiber, vitamins, and probiotics. This quinoa salad not only satisfies your hunger but also supports digestive health with its wholesome ingredients.

Lentil Soup

Ingredients:

1.   1 cup lentils (any color), rinsed

2.   1 onion, chopped

3.   2 carrots, diced

4.   2 celery stalks, diced

5.   4 cups vegetable broth

6.   1 teaspoon cumin

7.   Salt and pepper to taste

Instructions:

Begin by preparing the vegetables. Chop one onion, dice two carrots, and two celery stalks. In a large pot, heat a small amount of oil over medium heat and sauté the chopped onion, carrots, and celery until they are softened and the onion becomes translucent. This usually takes about 5-7 minutes. Rinse one cup of lentils under cold water to remove any debris or impurities, then add them to the pot.

Pour in four cups of vegetable broth, which serves as the base of the soup, providing depth and flavor. Add one teaspoon of cumin for a warm, earthy taste, and season with salt and pepper to your preference. Bring the mixture to a boil over high heat. Once boiling, reduce the heat to low and let the soup simmer for 25-30 minutes, or until the lentils are tender and fully cooked.

Throughout the cooking process, occasionally stir the soup to prevent the lentils from sticking to the bottom of the pot. Once the lentils are soft and the flavors have melded together, your soup is ready to serve. For an added touch, garnish the soup with fresh herbs like parsley or cilantro. This hearty lentil soup is not only comforting and delicious but also packed with protein, fiber, and essential nutrients, making it an ideal choice for a wholesome, satisfying lunch.

Dinner Recipes
Baked Salmon with Asparagus

This baked salmon recipe is a perfect choice for a healthy and delicious dinner. It features succulent salmon fillets paired with fresh asparagus, all baked to perfection with minimal effort.

Ingredients:

1. 2 salmon fillets

2. 1 bunch asparagus, trimmed

3. 2 tablespoons olive oil

4. 1 lemon, sliced

5. Salt and pepper to taste

Instructions:

1. Preheat the Oven: Start by preheating your oven to 400°F (200°C). This ensures that your salmon and asparagus cook evenly and come out tender and flavorful.

2. Prepare the Baking Sheet: Line a baking sheet with parchment paper for easy cleanup. Place the salmon fillets on

one side of the sheet and arrange the trimmed asparagus alongside them.

3.   Seasoning: Drizzle the olive oil over the salmon and asparagus, making sure to coat them well. Sprinkle salt and pepper to taste. This simple seasoning enhances the natural flavors of the ingredients.

4.   Add Lemon: Place lemon slices on top of each salmon fillet. The lemon adds a refreshing citrusy flavor that complements the richness of the salmon.

5.   Bake: Transfer the baking sheet to the preheated oven. Bake for 15-20 minutes, or until the salmon is cooked through and flakes easily with a fork. The asparagus should be tender yet crisp.

Stir-Fried Tofu with Broccoli

For those looking for a vegetarian option, this stir-fried tofu with broccoli is both satisfying and nutritious. It's a vibrant dish full of textures and flavors that can be prepared in under 30 minutes.

Ingredients:

1. 1 block firm tofu, cubed

2. 2 cups broccoli florets

3. 1 bell pepper, sliced

4. 2 cloves garlic, minced

5. 2 tablespoons soy sauce or tamari

6. Olive oil for frying

Instructions:

1. Heat the Oil: In a large pan, heat a tablespoon of olive oil over medium heat.

Once hot, add the minced garlic and sauté for about 1 minute until fragrant.

2.   Fry the Tofu: Add the cubed tofu to the pan. Fry until golden brown on all sides, about 5-7 minutes. This step is crucial for achieving a nice texture.

3.   Add Vegetables: Stir in the broccoli florets and sliced bell pepper. Cook for an additional 4-5 minutes until the vegetables are tender but still crisp.

4.   Flavor it Up: Pour in the soy sauce or tamari, stirring everything together. Cook for another minute, allowing the sauce to coat the tofu and vegetables evenly.

Snack Recipes
Apple Slices with Almond Butter

If you're looking for a quick and nutritious snack that satisfies your sweet tooth, try apple slices paired with almond butter. This simple yet delicious combination is not only easy to prepare but also packed with health benefits.

Ingredients:

1.   1 crisp apple (such as Fuji, Gala, or Granny Smith)

2.   2 tablespoons of almond butter

3.   A sprinkle of cinnamon (optional, but recommended)

Instructions:

1.   Begin by washing the apple thoroughly under running water to remove any dirt or residues. Once clean, slice the apple into wedges or rounds, depending on your preference. Aim for slices that are easy to dip and eat.

2.   Place the almond butter in a small bowl for easy dipping. The creamy texture of almond butter pairs perfectly with the crispness of the apple slices, creating a delightful contrast.

3.   For an added touch of flavor and health benefits, consider sprinkling a dash of cinnamon over the almond butter or directly onto the apple slices. Cinnamon not only enhances the taste but is also known for its anti-inflammatory properties and ability to help regulate blood sugar levels.

Vegetable Sticks with Hummus

For a savory snack that's equally nutritious, vegetable sticks with hummus are a fantastic option. This combination is not only colorful and appealing but also packed with vitamins, minerals, and fiber, making it an excellent choice for anyone looking to eat healthier.

Ingredients:

1.   Carrot sticks

2.   Cucumber sticks

3.   Bell pepper strips (red, yellow, or green)

4.   ½ cup of hummus for dipping

Instructions:

1.   Begin by washing your vegetables under cold water to ensure they are clean and fresh. Peel the carrots if desired, then cut them into sticks. Slice the cucumber into sticks or rounds, and cut the bell peppers into strips. Aim for uniform sizes for an appealing presentation.

2.   Arrange the prepared vegetable sticks artfully on a plate or a shallow bowl. This not only makes the snack visually appealing but also encourages healthy snacking, especially for kids.

3.   Serve the vegetable sticks alongside hummus in a small bowl. Hummus, made primarily from chickpeas, is rich in protein and fiber, providing a satisfying dip that complements the crunchiness of the vegetables. You can choose store-bought hummus or make your own by blending chickpeas, tahini, lemon juice, garlic, and olive oil.

Smoothies And Beverages

Incorporating smoothies and healthful beverages into your daily routine can be an enjoyable and nutritious way to enhance your overall well-being. Here, we'll explore two delicious recipes: a Green Gut Health Smoothie and a Ginger Turmeric Tea, both of which are not only easy to prepare but also packed with beneficial ingredients.

Green Gut Health Smoothie

This refreshing Green Gut Health Smoothie is perfect for a quick breakfast or an energizing snack. It combines nutrient-dense ingredients that support gut health and provide a burst of energy to kickstart your day.

Ingredients:

1.   1 cup spinach: Rich in vitamins A, C, and K, as well as iron and magnesium, spinach is an excellent leafy green that aids digestion.

2.   1 banana: Bananas add natural sweetness and are high in potassium, which helps maintain electrolyte balance.

3.   ½ avocado: Avocados contribute healthy fats that promote satiety and support heart health.

4.   1 cup almond milk: A dairy-free alternative, almond milk is low in calories and packed with vitamin E.

5.   1 tablespoon chia seeds: These tiny seeds are high in omega-3 fatty acids and fiber, promoting gut health and fullness.

Instructions:

1.   Combine all ingredients in a blender.

2.   Blend until smooth and creamy.

3. Serve immediately for a refreshing drink that nourishes your body and satisfies your taste buds.

The combination of these ingredients makes this smoothie not only delicious but also beneficial for gut health, ensuring you start your day on a healthy note.

Ginger Turmeric Tea

Next, we have the invigorating Ginger Turmeric Tea, a soothing beverage with anti-inflammatory properties. This tea is perfect for those chilly evenings or whenever you need a comforting drink.

Ingredients:

1. 2 cups water: The base for your tea.

2.   1 teaspoon fresh ginger, grated: Ginger is known for its anti-inflammatory and digestive benefits.

3.   1 teaspoon turmeric powder: Turmeric contains curcumin, which has potent anti-inflammatory properties and may help boost your immune system.

4.   Honey to taste (optional): Adding honey can enhance the flavor and provide additional soothing properties.

Instructions:

1.   Boil water in a saucepan.

2.   Add the grated ginger and turmeric powder to the boiling water.

3.   Simmer for 10 minutes to allow the flavors to meld, then strain into a cup.

4.   Add honey if desired and enjoy warm.

CHAPTER SIX

HEALING THE GUT

Identifying And Addressing Gut Issues

The first step in healing the gut begins with recognizing potential issues. Many individuals experience common signs of gut problems, such as bloating, gas, irregular bowel movements, fatigue, and food intolerances. These symptoms can significantly impact overall well-being and daily functioning. Therefore, it's essential to pay attention to these warning signals and take proactive steps toward understanding their root causes.

One effective method for identifying gut issues is to maintain a food diary. This involves documenting everything you eat and drink, along with any symptoms that arise afterward. By keeping track of your meals and corresponding reactions, you can begin to identify patterns that may point to specific foods or habits contributing to your discomfort. For example, you might notice that dairy products lead to bloating, or high-fiber foods cause irregular bowel movements. Such insights can be invaluable for determining which foods to eliminate or limit.

Once potential gut issues have been identified, the next crucial step is to address them. Consulting a healthcare professional is highly recommended, as they can guide you through appropriate tests and assessments. Conditions such as irritable bowel syndrome (IBS), celiac disease, or infections may require specialized diagnostic procedures. Early diagnosis is key, as it allows for more effective treatment options tailored to your specific needs.

Healthcare professionals may suggest various interventions based on your diagnosis. These could include dietary modifications, such as adopting a low-FODMAP diet for IBS or eliminating gluten for celiac disease. Probiotics may also be recommended to help restore gut flora balance. Additionally, lifestyle changes, such as increasing hydration, improving sleep quality, and managing stress, can have a significant positive impact on gut health.

Furthermore, it's essential to approach gut healing holistically. This means not only focusing on dietary changes but also considering the psychological and emotional aspects of health. Stress management techniques like mindfulness, yoga, or meditation can help reduce gut-related symptoms, as stress has been shown to influence gut function significantly.

Elimination Diets And Their Role

An elimination diet is an effective strategy for healing the gut, particularly for individuals experiencing food sensitivities or gastrointestinal issues. This dietary approach involves systematically removing common allergens and irritants from your diet for a designated period, typically lasting between four to six weeks. During this time, a variety of foods are eliminated, including gluten, dairy, soy, corn, and processed sugars. The goal is to give the gut a chance to heal and to reduce inflammation caused by potential dietary triggers.

The process begins with the complete removal of these foods, allowing for a period of detoxification. This phase helps identify how the body reacts when these irritants are absent. After the elimination period, foods are gradually reintroduced one at a time. This careful reintroduction helps observe any adverse reactions, making it easier to pinpoint specific food intolerances or sensitivities. For instance, after reintroducing dairy, an individual may notice symptoms such as bloating or digestive discomfort, indicating a potential sensitivity.

Elimination diets can provide numerous benefits beyond identifying food sensitivities. By reducing inflammation in the gut, they can alleviate symptoms associated with conditions like irritable bowel syndrome (IBS), bloating, and other digestive disturbances. This dietary approach also encourages individuals to become more mindful of their eating habits and the effects that various foods have on their overall health.

However, it's essential to approach elimination diets with caution and under the guidance of a healthcare professional. While the elimination diet can be beneficial, it may not be suitable for everyone. A healthcare provider can help tailor the diet to individual needs, ensuring that it is safe and effective. They can also monitor for potential nutritional deficiencies that may arise from eliminating entire food groups.

Supplements For Gut Health

Maintaining optimal gut health is essential for overall well-being, and while diet plays a crucial role, certain supplements can significantly aid in gut healing and function. Among these, probiotics and prebiotics are two key players that can help restore and support a balanced gut microbiome.

Probiotics are live beneficial bacteria that contribute to gut health by restoring the natural balance of flora in the digestive tract. These microorganisms can be found in fermented foods such as yogurt, kefir, sauerkraut, kimchi, and kombucha. Alternatively, they can be taken in the form of dietary supplements, available as capsules, tablets, or powders. Research has shown that probiotics can help alleviate symptoms of gastrointestinal disorders, particularly irritable bowel syndrome (IBS), which often manifests as bloating, gas, and irregular bowel movements. In addition to improving digestion, probiotics may also enhance the immune system, reduce inflammation, and contribute to mental health by impacting the gut-brain axis.

In contrast, prebiotics are non-digestible fibers that serve as food for probiotics, promoting their growth and activity within the gut. By nourishing beneficial bacteria, prebiotics help create an optimal environment for gut health. Foods that are rich in prebiotics include garlic, onions, leeks, asparagus, bananas, and whole grains. Incorporating these foods into your diet can stimulate the growth of healthy gut bacteria, leading to improved digestion and enhanced nutrient absorption.

The synergy between probiotics and prebiotics is particularly noteworthy. When consumed together, they can create a more robust gut ecosystem. This combination not only aids digestion but may also provide additional benefits, such as improved metabolism, increased resistance to infections, and enhanced mood. Some studies suggest that a healthy gut microbiome may even play a role in weight management and reducing the risk of chronic diseases, including diabetes and heart disease.

For individuals seeking to optimize their gut health, it's essential to consider both probiotics and prebiotics as part of a comprehensive approach. While dietary sources are an excellent way to obtain these supplements, some individuals may choose to incorporate high-quality supplements to ensure adequate intake. However, it's always advisable to consult with a healthcare professional before beginning any new supplement regimen, especially for those with existing health conditions or those taking medications.

The Role Of Hydration

Hydration plays a crucial yet often overlooked role in maintaining gut health. Water is fundamental for several digestive processes and overall well-being. It aids digestion by helping to break down food, making nutrients easier for the body to absorb. When we consume sufficient water, it assists in dissolving vitamins and minerals, facilitating their uptake by the intestines. This is particularly important because without adequate hydration, the digestive system can become sluggish, leading to various issues.

One of the most common consequences of dehydration is constipation. When the body lacks sufficient water, it absorbs more fluid from the waste material in the intestines, resulting in harder, more difficult-to-pass stools. This can create discomfort and disrupt regular bowel movements. Drinking enough water throughout the day is vital for softening stool and promoting healthy bowel habits. Experts recommend adjusting water intake based on factors such as physical activity, climate, and individual health needs to ensure optimal hydration.

In addition to plain water, other beverages can also contribute significantly to hydration. Herbal teas, for instance, offer both hydration and unique health benefits. Peppermint tea is renowned for its ability to soothe an upset stomach, providing relief from digestive discomfort and bloating. Ginger tea is another excellent option, known for its anti-nausea properties, making it particularly beneficial for those dealing with motion sickness or morning nausea. These herbal infusions not only enhance hydration but also offer additional support to gut health.

Broths, especially bone broth, are another excellent source of hydration. They provide not only fluids but also essential nutrients, including collagen and amino acids, which can support gut lining health and overall digestive function. Incorporating these hydrating options into your daily routine can enhance your overall health while providing a flavorful way to meet your hydration needs.

Detoxifying The Gut

Detoxifying the gut may sound daunting, but it can be a valuable practice for those dealing with persistent digestive issues. The goal of gut detoxification is to eliminate toxins from the digestive system, allowing it to function at its best. A gentle detox focuses on nourishing the body rather than imposing strict and often harsh protocols.

To start, incorporating whole, unprocessed foods into your diet is essential. These foods are not only nutrient-dense but also free from the additives and preservatives commonly found in processed options. Whole foods can enhance digestive health and support the body's natural detoxification processes. Emphasizing fruits, vegetables, whole grains, lean proteins, and healthy fats can provide the body with the necessary nutrients for optimal functioning.

Increasing fiber intake is another crucial aspect of gut detoxification. Fiber-rich foods, such as legumes, fruits, and vegetables, help promote regular bowel movements, which are vital for flushing out toxins. High-fiber foods also feed beneficial gut bacteria, contributing to a balanced gut microbiome. A healthy gut flora is essential for efficient digestion and overall health.

Certain foods have a particular reputation for supporting detoxification. Leafy greens, such as spinach and kale, are packed with vitamins and minerals that help combat oxidative stress. Cruciferous vegetables like broccoli, cauliflower, and Brussels sprouts contain compounds that support the liver, one of the body's primary detox organs. Additionally, fruits high in antioxidants, such as berries, can neutralize free radicals and reduce inflammation in the body.

Fermented foods also play a significant role in gut health and detoxification. Foods like yogurt, kefir, sauerkraut, and kimchi are rich in probiotics, which are beneficial bacteria that support a healthy gut flora. By enhancing gut flora diversity, these foods can improve digestion and bolster the body's natural detoxification mechanisms.

However, it is important to approach gut detoxification with caution. Extreme detox diets or cleanses can be overly aggressive and may lead to nutrient deficiencies or other health issues. Instead, focus on sustainable lifestyle changes that promote long-term health rather than quick fixes.

☐

CHAPTER SEVEN

LIFESTYLE CHANGES FOR A HEALTHY GUT

The Importance Of Physical Activity

Physical activity plays a crucial role in maintaining a healthy gut, offering numerous benefits that extend beyond digestive health to overall well-being. Regular exercise is a powerful stimulant for the digestive system, promoting the efficient movement of food through the intestines. This increased motility helps prevent common gastrointestinal issues such as constipation and bloating, ensuring a smoother and more comfortable digestive process.

One of the key benefits of physical activity on gut health is its impact on gut microbiota. The gut microbiome, which consists of trillions of bacteria, viruses, and fungi, plays an essential role in our overall health. Exercise has been shown to enhance the diversity and abundance of beneficial gut bacteria. A diverse microbiome is associated with better immune function, improved metabolism, and a lower risk of various diseases. The changes in gut microbiota induced by regular physical activity can lead to positive outcomes such as improved digestion, enhanced nutrient absorption, and a stronger immune system.

Engaging in at least 30 minutes of moderate exercise most days of the week can yield significant benefits for gut health. Activities such as walking, jogging, cycling, and swimming are excellent options. These forms of exercise are accessible and can be easily incorporated into daily routines. The key is consistency; regular physical activity ensures that the digestive system remains active and efficient.

Moreover, exercise has a direct impact on reducing inflammation in the body, including the gut. Chronic inflammation is a common underlying factor in many gastrointestinal disorders, including inflammatory bowel disease (IBD) and irritable bowel syndrome (IBS). By reducing inflammation, physical activity can alleviate symptoms and improve the quality of life for individuals with these conditions. Exercise also promotes better blood circulation, which ensures that the digestive organs receive an adequate supply of oxygen and nutrients, further supporting their function.

The benefits of physical activity extend beyond the gut, contributing to overall health and the prevention of chronic diseases. Regular exercise helps maintain a healthy weight, reducing the risk of obesity—a significant risk factor for various gastrointestinal issues and other chronic conditions such as diabetes and heart disease. Exercise also improves insulin sensitivity, which is crucial for metabolic health and preventing type 2 diabetes.

Furthermore, engaging in physical activity has positive effects on mental health. Stress and anxiety can negatively impact the gut, leading to symptoms such as indigestion and irritable bowel syndrome. Exercise is a natural stress reliever, promoting the release of endorphins and other neurotransmitters that enhance mood and reduce stress levels. This, in turn, can lead to improved gut health and a reduction in stress-related digestive issues.

Stress Management Techniques

Stress significantly impacts gut health, often leading to various gastrointestinal issues. When the body is under stress, it releases hormones such as cortisol, which can disrupt the balance of gut bacteria. This imbalance can result in problems like irritable bowel syndrome (IBS) and other digestive disorders. Therefore, managing stress effectively is crucial for maintaining a healthy gut and overall well-being.

One of the most effective stress management techniques is meditation. Regular meditation practice helps calm the mind and body, reducing the production of stress hormones. By focusing on breathing and mindfulness, meditation can lower blood pressure, decrease anxiety, and improve emotional health. Deep breathing exercises are another simple yet powerful tool for stress reduction. By consciously controlling your breath, you can activate the body's relaxation response, slowing the heart rate and promoting a sense of calm.

Yoga and tai chi are physical activities that combine movement with mindfulness, offering dual benefits for stress management and physical fitness. Yoga involves various postures and breathing techniques that help relax the body and mind. It also promotes flexibility and strength, contributing to overall physical health. Tai chi, often described as meditation in motion, involves slow, deliberate movements and deep breathing. It has been shown to reduce stress, improve balance, and enhance mental clarity.

Engaging in hobbies and activities you enjoy is another effective way to manage stress. Whether it's painting, gardening, reading, or playing a musical instrument, these activities can provide a much-needed distraction from daily stressors. They offer an opportunity to relax, recharge, and cultivate a sense of accomplishment and joy.

Spending time in nature has also been proven to reduce stress levels. Activities like hiking, walking in the park, or simply sitting by a lake can have a calming effect on the mind and body. Nature exposure can lower cortisol levels, reduce anxiety, and improve mood, contributing to better overall health.

Maintaining social connections is crucial for stress management. Positive relationships provide emotional support, reduce feelings of isolation, and enhance well-being. Whether through family, friends, or community groups, social interactions can help buffer the effects of stress and provide a sense of belonging and security.

Sleep Hygiene And Gut Health

Good sleep hygiene is essential for maintaining a healthy gut. The intricate relationship between sleep and gut health is becoming increasingly clear through scientific research. Poor sleep can disrupt the balance of gut bacteria and increase inflammation, leading to various digestive issues. Understanding and improving sleep hygiene can significantly enhance gut health and overall well-being.

To begin with, establishing a regular sleep schedule is crucial. Going to bed and waking up at the same time each day helps regulate the body's internal clock, also known as the circadian rhythm. Consistency in sleep patterns allows the body to anticipate and prepare for rest, promoting more profound and more restorative sleep. This, in turn, positively influences the gut microbiome by maintaining a stable environment for beneficial bacteria to thrive.

Creating a relaxing bedtime routine is another vital aspect of good sleep hygiene. Engaging in calming activities before bed can signal to the body that it is time to wind down. Reading a book, taking a warm bath, or practicing relaxation exercises such as deep breathing, meditation, or gentle yoga can help ease the mind and body into a state conducive to sleep. These activities reduce stress and anxiety, which are known to negatively impact gut health by altering the balance of gut bacteria and increasing inflammation.

The sleep environment itself plays a significant role in promoting quality sleep. Ensuring that your bedroom is comfortable, cool, and free from distractions can make a substantial difference. A quiet, dark, and cool room creates an optimal environment for sleep. Investing in a good mattress and pillows can also enhance comfort and support better sleep posture, reducing the likelihood of waking up with aches and pains that could disturb sleep continuity.

Limiting exposure to screens before bedtime is another critical factor. The blue light emitted by phones, tablets, computers, and televisions can interfere with the production of melatonin, the hormone responsible for regulating sleep-wake cycles. Reducing screen time at least an hour before bed can help mitigate this effect and promote better sleep.

Additionally, avoiding caffeine and heavy meals close to bedtime is essential. Caffeine is a stimulant that can keep you awake, while heavy meals can cause discomfort and indigestion, disrupting sleep. Opting for light snacks if needed and ensuring that the last meal of the day is consumed at least a few hours before bedtime can support better sleep quality.

Adequate sleep supports the body's natural repair processes and promotes a healthy gut microbiome. During sleep, the body undergoes essential restorative processes, including the repair of tissues, the strengthening of the immune system, and the regulation of hormones. These processes are crucial for maintaining a balanced and healthy gut microbiome. Conversely, chronic sleep deprivation can lead to dysbiosis, an imbalance in the gut bacteria, contributing to various health issues, including digestive problems, obesity, and even mental health disorders.

Mindful Eating Practices

Mindful eating is a practice that involves paying full attention to the eating experience, which can greatly benefit gut health. This approach encourages you to eat slowly and savor each bite, allowing your digestive system to process food more efficiently. As a result, mindful eating can help prevent overeating, reduce symptoms of indigestion, and improve nutrient absorption, all of which are crucial for maintaining a healthy gut.

One of the key principles of mindful eating is eliminating distractions during meals. This means turning off the TV, putting away your phone, and creating a calm, focused environment where you can fully engage with your food. By doing so, you can concentrate on the sensory experience of eating, noticing the taste, texture, and aroma of each bite. This heightened awareness not only enhances the enjoyment of food but also promotes better digestion. When you eat without distractions, you are more likely to chew your food thoroughly, which is the first step in the digestive process. Chewing breaks down food into smaller pieces, making it easier for your stomach and intestines to digest and absorb nutrients.

Another important aspect of mindful eating is listening to your body's hunger and fullness cues. Often, people eat out of habit, boredom, or emotional triggers, rather than true hunger. Mindful eating encourages you to pause and assess whether you are genuinely hungry before reaching for food. This practice helps regulate food intake and prevents overeating, which can lead to digestive discomfort and weight gain. By paying attention to your body's signals, you can eat in response to physical hunger and stop when you feel satisfied, rather than continuing to eat until you are overly full.

Mindful eating also involves appreciating the journey of your food from its source to your plate. This awareness can foster a greater appreciation for the food you eat and the effort that goes into producing it. Taking the time to think about where your food comes from and how it was prepared can enhance your connection to your meals and promote a more balanced and respectful relationship with food.

Practicing mindful eating can have profound benefits for your gut health. By eating slowly and without distractions, you give your digestive system the time it needs to effectively process food. Chewing thoroughly aids in breaking down food, which improves nutrient absorption and reduces the likelihood of indigestion. Additionally, by listening to your body's hunger and fullness cues, you can avoid overeating and maintain a healthy weight, further supporting gut health. Overall, mindful eating encourages a more thoughtful and conscious approach to eating that can lead to improved digestion, better nutrient absorption, and a healthier relationship with food.

Long-Term Strategies For Maintaining Gut Health

Maintaining gut health is essential for overall well-being, requiring a long-term commitment to lifestyle changes and healthy habits. Central to this is a balanced diet that promotes a diverse and thriving gut microbiome. Consuming a variety of fiber-rich foods, such as fruits, vegetables, whole grains, legumes, and nuts, is crucial. Fiber acts as a prebiotic, feeding beneficial bacteria in the gut and aiding in digestion. Incorporating fermented foods like yogurt, kefir, sauerkraut, kimchi, and miso introduces probiotics, which are live beneficial bacteria that can help balance the gut microbiome.

Hydration also plays a significant role in maintaining gut health. Drinking plenty of water helps with digestion and supports the mucosal lining of the intestines, which serves as a barrier against harmful substances. Proper hydration ensures that the digestive system functions smoothly, preventing issues such as constipation.

Regular physical activity is another critical factor in promoting gut health. Exercise stimulates the muscles in the gastrointestinal tract, aiding in the movement of food through the digestive system and reducing the risk of constipation. It also helps reduce inflammation, a common issue that can negatively impact gut health. Additionally, physical activity can contribute to maintaining a healthy weight, which is linked to a lower risk of developing conditions such as irritable bowel syndrome (IBS) and gastroesophageal reflux disease (GERD).

Stress management is equally important for gut health. Chronic stress can disrupt the balance of bacteria in the gut, leading to digestive issues. Practices such as mindfulness, meditation, yoga, and deep-breathing exercises can help manage stress levels and support a healthy gut-brain connection.

Good sleep hygiene is essential for maintaining gut health. Poor sleep patterns can disrupt the gut microbiome, leading to imbalances that can affect digestion and overall health. Aim for 7-9 hours of quality sleep per night to support your gut health.

Avoiding smoking and limiting alcohol consumption are also vital strategies for gut health. Smoking can damage the gut lining and alter the gut microbiome, leading to an increased risk of gastrointestinal diseases. Similarly, excessive alcohol consumption can cause inflammation and harm the gut lining, disrupting the balance of gut bacteria.

In addition to dietary and lifestyle changes, incorporating supplements like probiotics and prebiotics can be beneficial. Probiotics, found in supplements and fermented foods, introduce beneficial bacteria to the gut. Prebiotics, found in foods such as garlic, onions, leeks, and bananas, provide nourishment for these beneficial bacteria, supporting their growth and activity.

Consistency in these practices is key to long-term gut health. By adopting a holistic approach that includes a balanced diet, regular exercise, stress management, good sleep hygiene, and avoiding harmful habits, you can maintain a healthy gut and improve your overall well-being.

CHAPTER EIGHT

SPECIAL CONSIDERATIONS

Gut Health During Pregnancy

Pregnancy is a pivotal period that significantly influences the health of both the mother and the developing baby, making gut health a critical focus. Hormonal fluctuations, dietary changes, and the physical demands of the growing fetus can all impact the digestive system, leading to common issues such as constipation and heartburn. Addressing these concerns through proper diet, hydration, probiotics, and exercise can greatly benefit overall digestive health during pregnancy.

One of the primary digestive issues faced by pregnant women is constipation. Hormonal changes, particularly the increase in progesterone, can slow down the movement of food through the digestive tract. Additionally, the growing uterus can put pressure on the intestines, further exacerbating the problem. To alleviate constipation, it is essential to consume a diet rich in fiber. Fiber adds bulk to the stool and helps it move more easily through the digestive system. Good sources of dietary fiber include fruits, vegetables, and whole grains. For example, incorporating foods like apples, berries, carrots, broccoli, oats, and brown rice into daily meals can provide the necessary fiber intake.

Hydration is another crucial factor in maintaining gut health during pregnancy. Drinking plenty of water helps soften the stool and promotes regular bowel movements. It is recommended that pregnant women drink at least eight to ten glasses of water a day. This not only aids digestion but also helps prevent dehydration, which can contribute to other pregnancy-related issues such as headaches and fatigue.

Probiotics play a significant role in maintaining a healthy balance of gut bacteria. These beneficial microorganisms can be found in supplements and fermented foods such as yogurt, kefir, sauerkraut, and kimchi. Probiotics help enhance digestion and support the immune system, which is particularly important during pregnancy when the body's immune response is naturally altered. Regular consumption of probiotic-rich foods can help mitigate digestive discomfort and promote a healthy gut environment for both the mother and the developing baby.

Heartburn is another common digestive complaint during pregnancy, often caused by the relaxation of the lower esophageal sphincter due to hormonal changes. To manage heartburn, pregnant women should avoid large, fatty meals and instead opt for smaller, more frequent meals throughout the day. It is also advisable to avoid lying down immediately after eating and to elevate the head while sleeping to prevent stomach acid from rising.

In addition to dietary adjustments, regular, gentle exercise can significantly contribute to healthy digestion. Activities such as walking, swimming, and prenatal yoga can stimulate intestinal activity and promote overall well-being. Exercise also helps manage weight gain and reduces the risk of gestational diabetes and hypertension, further supporting a healthy pregnancy.

By focusing on a balanced diet rich in fiber, staying well-hydrated, incorporating probiotics, and engaging in regular exercise, pregnant women can effectively manage digestive issues and maintain optimal gut health. This holistic approach not only enhances the mother's well-being but also supports the healthy development of the baby.

Children's Gut Health

Children's gut health is foundational for their overall growth and development. A well-balanced diet rich in diverse nutrients plays a crucial role in fostering a healthy gut microbiome in children. The gut microbiome, a complex community of microorganisms living in the digestive tract, significantly impacts digestion, immune function, and even brain development. By introducing a variety of fruits, vegetables, whole grains, and fermented foods early on, parents can help establish a robust and diverse gut microbiota in their children.

Fruits and vegetables are excellent sources of fiber, vitamins, and minerals, which are essential for the growth of beneficial gut bacteria. Whole grains, such as oats, brown rice, and whole wheat, provide additional fiber and nutrients that support a healthy digestive system. Fermented foods like yogurt, kefir, sauerkraut, and miso contain probiotics, which are live beneficial bacteria that can enhance gut health. Including these foods in a child's diet can promote a balanced gut microbiome and improve overall health.

It is also important to limit the intake of processed foods and sugary snacks, which can negatively impact gut health. Processed foods often contain artificial additives, preservatives, and high levels of sugar and unhealthy fats, all of which can disrupt the balance of gut bacteria. Sugary snacks can lead to the growth of harmful bacteria and yeast in the gut, potentially causing digestive issues and weakening the immune system.

For children who experience digestive issues like constipation or diarrhea, natural remedies can be particularly effective. Increasing fiber intake through fruits, vegetables, and whole grains can help regulate bowel movements and alleviate constipation. Incorporating probiotics through fermented foods or supplements can help restore the balance of gut bacteria, improving symptoms of diarrhea and other digestive problems. Additionally, staying hydrated by drinking plenty of water is essential for maintaining healthy digestion and preventing constipation.

Parents should also be mindful of antibiotic use, as these medications can disrupt the gut microbiome by killing not only harmful bacteria but also beneficial ones. While antibiotics are sometimes necessary to treat bacterial infections, their overuse or misuse can have long-term negative effects on gut health. When antibiotics are prescribed, it is important to follow the healthcare provider's instructions carefully and consider using probiotics to help restore the gut microbiome after the treatment.

Supporting children's gut health through proper nutrition and lifestyle habits is an investment in their future well-being. By fostering a diverse and balanced gut microbiome, parents can help their children develop a strong immune system, better digestion, and even improved cognitive function. Emphasizing the importance of a healthy diet, regular physical activity, and mindful antibiotic use can set children up for a healthier and happier life.

Gut Health For Seniors

As we age, maintaining gut health becomes increasingly crucial due to the natural changes that occur in the digestive system. Seniors often face a slowdown in digestive processes, which can lead to common issues such as constipation and reduced nutrient absorption. Understanding and addressing these changes through diet and lifestyle modifications is essential for promoting overall well-being in older adults.

One of the primary dietary focuses for seniors should be on increasing fiber intake. A high-fiber diet helps in maintaining regular bowel movements and preventing constipation, a common issue among the elderly. Incorporating plenty of fruits, vegetables, legumes, and whole grains can significantly enhance fiber intake. Foods such as berries, apples, carrots, beans, and oats are excellent sources of dietary fiber. By making these foods a staple in their diet, seniors can support smoother digestive processes and better nutrient absorption.

Staying hydrated is equally important. Dehydration can exacerbate constipation and contribute to other digestive discomforts. Seniors should aim to drink plenty of water throughout the day. Herbal teas, clear soups, and water-rich fruits like watermelon and cucumber can also contribute to overall hydration. Keeping a regular schedule for fluid intake, especially if there are concerns about forgetting to drink water, can help seniors stay adequately hydrated.

In addition to fiber and hydration, probiotics and prebiotics play a vital role in maintaining gut health. Probiotics are beneficial bacteria that help balance the gut microbiome, and they can be found in foods like yogurt, kefir, sauerkraut, and other fermented products. Prebiotics, on the other hand, are non-digestible fibers that feed these beneficial bacteria, promoting their growth and activity. Foods like asparagus, garlic, onions, and bananas are rich in prebiotics. Seniors can also consider taking probiotic and prebiotic supplements after consulting with healthcare providers to ensure they are appropriate for their individual health needs.

Regular physical activity is another critical factor in promoting gut health for seniors. Exercise stimulates intestinal contractions, which can help prevent constipation and improve overall digestive function. Activities such as walking, swimming, and yoga are gentle on the joints and can be easily integrated into a daily routine. Even light physical activity can make a significant difference in maintaining a healthy digestive system.

Medications can also impact gut health. Many commonly prescribed drugs for seniors, such as pain relievers, antacids, and certain blood pressure medications, can disrupt the digestive system. It is essential for seniors to discuss their medications with healthcare providers, exploring gut-friendly alternatives if necessary. Adjustments in medication or the introduction of supplements to counteract negative digestive effects can help mitigate these issues.

Managing Gut Health With Chronic Illnesses

Chronic illnesses such as diabetes, irritable bowel syndrome (IBS), and inflammatory bowel disease (IBD) can profoundly impact gut health, requiring tailored approaches to diet and lifestyle to manage effectively. These conditions often necessitate specific dietary modifications to ensure optimal gut function and overall health.

For individuals with diabetes, managing blood sugar levels is paramount. A balanced diet rich in high-fiber foods can significantly benefit gut health. High-fiber foods help regulate blood sugar levels and promote healthy digestion, reducing the risk of complications. Including whole grains, fruits, vegetables, and legumes in the diet can enhance gut microbiota diversity, fostering a healthier gut environment. Regular monitoring of blood sugar levels combined with these dietary changes can lead to better management of diabetes and improved gut health.

 Managing IBS and IBD often involves identifying and avoiding trigger foods that exacerbate symptoms. These conditions can cause various digestive issues, such as bloating, abdominal pain, and irregular bowel movements. Foods high in FODMAPs (fermentable oligosaccharides, disaccharides, monosaccharides, and polyols) are common triggers for IBS symptoms. A low FODMAP diet, which involves eliminating high FODMAP foods and gradually reintroducing them to identify specific triggers, can be effective in managing symptoms. Individuals with IBD might benefit from an anti-inflammatory diet, focusing on reducing foods that can cause intestinal inflammation.

Collaborating with a dietitian is often beneficial for individuals with chronic illnesses. A dietitian can provide personalized nutrition plans tailored to individual needs and medical conditions. They can help identify trigger foods, suggest appropriate dietary adjustments, and ensure that nutritional needs are met. This professional guidance can be crucial in navigating the complex dietary requirements of chronic illnesses.

In addition to dietary changes, stress management plays a significant role in maintaining gut health. Chronic stress can negatively impact the gut-brain axis, exacerbating symptoms of IBS and IBD. Incorporating stress-reducing practices such as mindfulness, yoga, and regular exercise can improve gut health and overall well-being. These activities promote relaxation, reduce inflammation, and enhance the gut microbiota, contributing to better digestive health.

Probiotics are another tool that can support gut health in individuals with chronic illnesses. These beneficial bacteria can help balance the gut microbiome, reduce inflammation, and improve symptoms of digestive disorders. Incorporating probiotic-rich foods like yogurt, kefir, and fermented vegetables or taking probiotic supplements can be advantageous.

Understanding Food Sensitivities And Allergies

Food sensitivities and allergies can have a profound impact on digestive health and overall well-being. Both conditions can lead to significant discomfort and a variety of symptoms, such as bloating, gas, abdominal pain, and fatigue. Recognizing and avoiding trigger foods is essential for managing these symptoms and maintaining optimal gut health.

Food allergies are immune responses to certain proteins in foods, which can lead to severe reactions in some individuals. Common allergens include dairy, gluten, nuts, shellfish, eggs, and soy. Even a small amount of these foods can trigger reactions, which can range from mild symptoms like hives or stomach upset to life-threatening conditions such as anaphylaxis. For those with diagnosed food allergies, it is critical to read food labels carefully and be vigilant about cross-contamination.

On the other hand, food sensitivities do not involve the immune system but rather the digestive system's inability to properly process certain foods. This can lead to symptoms such as bloating, gas, and changes in bowel habits. Lactose intolerance is a well-known example, where individuals have difficulty digesting lactose, the sugar found in milk and dairy products. Other common sensitivities involve fructose, histamine, and certain artificial additives, which can trigger discomfort in susceptible individuals.

To effectively manage food sensitivities and allergies, keeping a detailed food diary can be highly beneficial. This practice allows individuals to track their food intake and any corresponding symptoms, helping to identify problematic foods. Once trigger foods are pinpointed, the next step is to eliminate them from the diet. However, it is equally important to find suitable alternatives to ensure that nutritional needs are met. For example, lactose-free dairy products or gluten-free grains can provide similar textures and flavors without triggering symptoms.

For individuals with severe food allergies, developing an action plan is vital. This plan should outline steps to take in the event of accidental exposure, including carrying an epinephrine auto-injector if prescribed. Education about food allergies and communication with family, friends, and restaurants about dietary restrictions can also help prevent exposure.

Working with a healthcare provider or a registered dietitian can provide valuable guidance in navigating food sensitivities and allergies. They can assist in creating a safe and effective eating plan that supports gut health while avoiding allergens and sensitivities. By understanding and managing these dietary issues, individuals can improve their quality of life and maintain better overall health.

THE END